Shinsei Mu Sool
Student Syllabus

By

Rev. Joshua D. Goepfrich

ISBN-13: 978-1516860661
ISBN-10: 1516860667

All exercise should be done carefully, with thought and
under a physician's approval

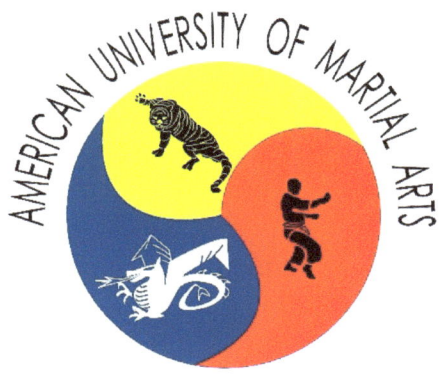

"Practical Values for Practical People"

Dear student,

Welcome to the American University of Martial Arts (AUMA). I would like to take a moment to express my deep desire to see each of you grow, not only as a martial artist, but as a spiritual warrior as well. When each of us realizes the potential our bodies have to offer we can exclaim as David did, "I thank you, High God – you're breathtaking! Body and soul, I am marvelously made! I worship in adoration – what a creation!" (Msg)

To understand the creation is to get to know the Creator. Let each of us take the opportunity to be good stewards of the bodies God has given to us. Our corporeal flesh will one day turn to dust, but to be able to worship God and show our adoration to Him through the life He has given to us is one of the purposes He has placed us here for.

Part of the beauty in this path that we have taken is the opportunity to visit another culture and through the outlook of other's eyes, see the way God is in control of all things. We would like to offer to you, our colleagues, the opportunity to come with us on our *Korean Cultural Tour*. Visit the site of ancient culture and experience the difference this makes in your life.

In order that you might be more prepared to train oversees, we have available for you to purchase our DVD series. This series includes all AUMA techniques from the manual as well as valuable information that will deepen your knowledge of God through the arts that we practice.

It is our job to pass Christian values on to others. My wife and I have decided to do this through martial technique. May we all set the standard for what a Christian martial artist should be.

May the Spirit of Christ dwell in you richly,

Master Joshua D. Goepfrich
President and Founder – AUMA

About this manual:

In this manual you, as a color belt student of the American University of Martial Arts, will have all the technical information you need to be able to test for your tips and belt ranks. However, this manual will not have every bit of information and cannot take the place of class instruction. Without proper instruction from a qualified AUMA instructor you may cause injury to yourself and others.

All students are required to learn the CREED as well as know all material previously learned.

Each belt rank has some information in bold type. These items will be the information that you are required to know to gain your tip. The rest of the information for that rank as well as the tip information is required to gain your next belt level.

Basic Terminology:

1	Hana		6	Yasut
2	Dul		7	Ilgop
3	Set		8	Yadool
4	Net		9	Ahope
5	Dasut		10	Yul
			20	Smool
			30	Sarahn

Always answer "Yes, sir (ma'am) or No, sir (ma'am) when talking to an instructor.

Our Creed: *Live by the Creed!!*

HONOR, RESPECT, COURAGE, LOYALTY, HUMILITY, PATIENCE, SELF-CONTROL

"The man who really wants to do something finds a way,
the other kind finds an excuse"

Stretching:

It is always important to make sure as you are stretching that your back is as straight as possible. Many people will try to stretch each muscle but twist their back at the same time to "reduce the stress on it." This type of "stretching" will compromise what each stretch is designed to accomplish because you are not letting the muscle work to its fullest potential.

The other main point to remember is that the muscles need to be relaxed and warm before extended stretching is possible. Light stretches at the beginning of a workout will help the muscles warm up. It is better to stretch the joints and ligaments at the beginning of the workout and the muscles after the first cardio warm-up.

The following list will help you remember each area that needs to be stretched properly for a complete body stretch:

Neck	Shoulders	Arms	Chest
Trunk	Sides	Hips	Upper Body
Knees	Back	Groin	Quadriceps
Hamstrings	Calf	Ankles	Appendages

Order of Class:

When you enter into the kwan: bow and remove shoes
Arrive ten minutes before class begins
Enter the dojang from the furthest outside edge – salute the flag
Uniform and belt must be worn at all times
Stretch and prepare body and mind for class
Mun yun prior to class
When prompted by instructor, rise into attention position
      Live by the Creed
Bow to flag/hand over heart
Bow to kwanjang – salute – dan kio
Bow to sabum – salute
Bow to instructors – salute
Il shim
Warm up with gibon and pal chaggi
Once class begins every student is expected to stay in it and do everything asked. There is no other option. (It is understood that illness and injury exist – if you do not feel well let the instructor know before class begins.) It does not matter whether what the instructor asks is possible or whether a student feels like doing a particular skill or drill. The only proper response is yes sir or yes ma'am.
In joining class a student agrees to be taught. To do otherwise is disrespect.

Warm – Up
Leadership class

- stretching should be done since been in more classes already
- Leadership quote
- Gibons and Pal Chaggis
- ½ mile run
- 20 pushups
- 10 forearm drills

Advance class

- stretching should be done since been in more classes already
- Leadership quote
- Gibons and Pal Chaggis
- Stairs with kicks
- 20 pushups
- Foot drills

Order will be maintained at all times. (See rules of the dojang) It is our intent to have a good God-honoring time while working out. If you have any questions please see your instructor.

The steps of a wise man are purposeful.

명예

전중하다

배짱

정절

비하

인내

자제

Notes

강설:

Meaning: Empty, looking to be filled
            Lack of color = innocence, purity
            Accepting new knowledge, embracing traditional values

Stretches
Order of Class
Creed of life
Mun Yun (calm the mind)
Insa (Etiquette)
Naup-Po (Falls)

One-steps: 1-3
Self-defense: attack from front

Gibon Hana   (Basic 1)   Pal Chaggi Hana (Kick drill 1)

Tae Geuk   **El-Jong**   Ee-Jong

Strikes -   **Chi-gi to solo plexus and injung (punch)**

Blocks –   **Ahn momtong maggi (inside body block)**
               Eolgul maggi (high block)
               Ahre maggi (low block)

Kicks -   **Ahp chaggi to solo plexus (front snap kick)**
               Yop chaggi to knee (side kick)
               Dolryo chaggi to knee (round kick)
               Naeryo chaggi (ax kick)
               Bakkat Bandouble chaggi (outer crescent kick)

Stances -   **Cha-ryot   (attention)**
               Pyong-hi sogi (ready stance)
               Juchoom sogi (horse stance)
               Ahp-gubi sogi (forward/front stance)
               Ahp-sogi (walking stance)
               Kyorugi sogi (fighting stance)

Terminology

Count 1 – 10	Dojang – gymnasium
Sabunim – master instructor	Joon bi - ready
Gamsahamnida – thank you	Ki hap - yell
Il shim – one heart	Charyot - attention
Poomse – moving meditation (forms)	Dan Kio – Teamwork
Kyong-ye – bow	Dobok – uniform

— Responsible for all previous material

Notes

Yellow Belt

Meaning: Sunrise or dawning of knowledge

One-steps: 4-6
Self-defense: front/rear
Power Check

Gibon Hana   Pal Chaggi Hana

Tae Guek   **Sam Jong**   Sa Jong

Strikes -   **Sonnal Chi-gi (knife strike)**
Jaebipoom mok chi-gi (high knife block & knife strike)
Dung-joomock chi-gi (back fist strike)

Blocks -   **Sonnal maggi (knife block - single** & double)

Kicks -   Yop chaggi to solo plexus (side kick)
Dolryo chaggi to solo plexus (round kick)
Ahn bandouble chaggi to shoulder height (inside crescent kick)
Ahp-jillo chaggi to solo plexus (thrusting kick)

Stances -   **Dwi-gibi sogi (back stance)**

Terminology

Dee – belt	Chiggi – strike
Maggi – block	Chaggi - kick
Dolryo – round	Dwi - back
Momtong – body	Barro - return
Eolgul – head	

— Responsible for all previous material

Notes

Meaning: Sky, Heaven
Ambition and deep desire for complexity and technique
Humility and patience

One-steps: 7-10
Self-defense: ground/side
Power check

Gibon Dul (Basic 2)   Pal Chaggi Dul (Kick drill 2)

Tae Geuk   **Oh-Jong**   Yook-Jong

Strikes -   Me-joomok chi-gi (hammer fist)
               Palkoop chi-gi (elbow strike)
               Pyon son-kut chi-gi (spear hand strike)

Blocks -   **Yeot pero maggi (X block)**
               Patang-son maggi (palm block)
               Badangson momtong nullo maggi (pressing down block)
               Bakkat momtong maggi (outer block)
               Pakhag momtong maggi (reverse outer block)

Kicks -   Twi (jumping):
               ahp chaggi
               dolryo chaggi
               yop chaggi
               backkat bandouble chaggi
               naeryo chaggi
               ahn bandouble chaggi
               back spin yop chaggi (turning side kick)
               moon thrust (crossing low kick)

Stances -   **Koa sogi (twisted stance)**

Terminology

Bakkat – outer   Kwanjangnim – grand master
Ahp – front   Seon bae – senior
Ahre – down   Kyosanim – black belt instructor
Twi – jump   Gu mahn – stop
Si-jak – begin

— Responsible for all previous material

Notes

Meaning: Mountains, earth
Firm foundation

One-steps: 11-13
Self-defense: 2 attackers
Power check
Required technique

Gibon Set (Basic 3)   Pal Chaggi Set (Kick drill 3)

Tae Geuk   **Chil-Jong**   Pal Jong

Strikes -   **Double upper cut**
                Sonnal-dung chi-gi (ridge hand strike)

Blocks -   Double ahre magi (two low blocks simultaneously)
                Kawi-u maggi (scissors block)
                Hecho maggi (spreading block)

Kicks -   **Guligi chaggi (hook kick to knee — to solo plexus and head)**
                Twi back spin yop chaggi (turning jump side kick)
                Moo-rup chaggi (knee kick)
                Skipping:
                          Ahp chaggi
                          Yop chaggi
                          Dolryo chaggi
                          Backkat bandouble chaggi
                          Ahn bandouble chaggi
                          Naeryo chaggi

Stances -   **Bum sogi (tiger stance)**
                Ryong sogi (dragon stance)

Terminology
                Injung – top of lip   Ahp-chook – ball of foot
                Left – left   Ahn - inner
                Right – right   Yop – side

— Responsible for all previous material

Notes

Meaning: Fire, sun = danger
Familiar with techniques, but still lacks necessary control to execute wisely in practice

One-steps: 1-13
Self-defense: ground 2 attackers
Power Check
Required technique

Gibon Hana, Dul, Set   Pal Chaggi Hana, Dul, Set

Tae Geuk   **All**

Strikes -   **Huryo chi-gi (hook punch)**
Uppercut
Ap-joomok chirugi (jab punch)
Reverse punch (counterpunch)

Blocks -   **All**

Kicks -   Dwi chaggi (back kick)
Back spin guligi chaggi (turning hook kick)

Stances -   **All**

Terminology
Kyorugi – sparring   Hosinsool – self-defense
Ba-quo – switch   Jochyo – junior

— Responsible for all previous material

Notes

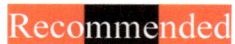

Meaning: Candidate for black belt

One-steps: 1-13
Self-defense: front/rear/sides/ground/multiple attacks
Power Check
Required technique

Gibon Hana, Dul, Set, Net   Pal Chaggi Hana, Dul, Set

Tae Geuk   **All**   Koryo

Strikes -   Agwi-son chi-gi (arc hand strike)
                Batang-son chi-gi (palm-heel strike)

Blocks -   Koryo

Kicks -   **Narabam (tornado roundhouse)**
                Ye tan chaggi (flying kick)

Stances -   Po jumok sogi (containing the vital energy stance)

Terminology
                All

— Responsible for all previous material

Notes

유술

White sash

Meaning: snow, without life but with potential
              (Spiritually – dead & without Christ)

Tiger One Steps 1-3
Dragon One Steps 1-3

Balance – Lift one foot slightly off the ground keeping leg straight and hold for 30+ sec

Pilates -   Frog
              Double Leg Lift 1
              Criss Cross
              Sliding Leg 1
              Hundred 1
              Pilates Pushup 1
              Single Leg Circles 1
              Front/Back

Stretches -   Warm up Stretch with Knee Sway
              Spinal Twist 1
              Cat Stretch 1
              Hip/Buttock Stretch
              Double Leg Stretch
              Single Leg Stretch 1
              Total Rest Pose
              Hip Opener 1
              Waist Twist
              Shoulder Roll
              Triceps Stretch
              Hip Circles

Millennium Exercise

Shepherd's Kata

Meditation – Proper Posture
       "I am fearfully and wonderfully made"

Notes

  Meaning: Movement begins with sunshine, morning
        (Spiritually – Christ is the Light of the World, brings new life)

Tiger One Steps – 4 – 6
Dragon One Steps – 4 – 6

Balance – Lift leg in front of body with knee bent at 90° and hold for 30+ sec

Pilates –   Hundred 2
      Bridge 1
      Side Leg Circles 1
      Side Leg Lift 1
      Single Leg Circles 2
      Pilates Push Up 2
      Double Leg Lift 2

Stretches -   Single Leg Stretch 2
      Spine Stretch Forward
      Spinal Twist 2
      Full Body Reach-Up
      Abdominal Lengthener
      One Leg Lift
      Back Strengthener
      Hamstring and Back Stretch Sequence 1

Weights -   Zip-Up
      Strong Man
      Side Raise
      Alternating Arms

Guryong Il Hang gu pyon

yuchea urlcheawee 유체 울체의 (fluid motion) 1-20

Meditation – Proper Breathing

Notes

Meaning: Begins to look more natural or filled out
(Spiritually – fruit begins to show)

Tiger One Steps 7-9
Dragon One Steps 7-9

Balance – Lift leg and bend knee so that knee is facing outward from body and lifted foot
          is level with straight knee. Hold for 30+ sec

Pilates -   Corkscrew
Can-Can 1
Leg Pull Front 1
Leg Pull Back
Bridge 2
Leg Lift with Reach 1
Sliding Leg 2
Lower Ab Strengthener 1
Roll-Up 1
Roll Down 1

Stretches -   Chest Expansion
Chest Opener
Leg Stretch
Lower Body Stretch
Neck-Shoulder-Back Relaxer
Buttocks Stretch 1

Weights: Ladybug
Arm Extension
Triceps Toner

Band: Hip and Outer Thigh Slimmer
Buttocks Firmer

Guryong Ee Hang gu pyon

yuchea urlcheawee 유체 울체의 (fluid motion) 21-30

Meditation – Proper Mind Set
          "I can do all things…"

Notes

Meaning: Water; deeper fluid motion; more understanding
(Spiritually – life flowing to others moving them to Christ)

Tiger One Steps 7-9
Dragon One Steps 7-9

Balance – Lift leg in front of body so that bent knee is at hip level and hold for 30+ sec

Pilates -
- Single Leg Circles 3
- Side Leg Circles 2
- Side Leg Lift 2
- One Leg Lift
- Plank 1
- Ab Lift
- The Saw
- Ab Curl 1
- Ab Strengthener

Stretches -
- Buttock Stretch 2
- Calf Stretch
- Thigh Stretch
- Triangle
- Hip Opener 2
- Cat Stretch 2
- Back and Hamstring Stretch 2
- Lower and Upper Back Strengthener
- Childs Pose

Weights:
- Double Arm Row
- One Arm Row
- Overhead Press

Band:
- Hamstring Curl
- Quad Firmer

Guryong Sam Hang gu pyon

yuchea urlcheawee 유체 울체의 (fluid motion) 31-40

Meditation – Proper Balance

Notes

Meaning: Blending of knowledge
(Spiritually – recognizing royal heritage in God our Father)

Tiger One Steps 10-11
Dragon One Steps 10-11

Balance – Lift leg so that bent knee is facing outward from body and lifted foot is barely touching the inner thigh of the straight leg and hold for 30+ sec.

Pilates -
Leg Pull Front 2
Bun Lifter
Bottom Firmer Sequence
Leg Beats
Inner Thigh Firmer
Super Woman
Swimming
Lower Ab Strengthener 2
Hundred 3
Roll-Up 2
Roll Down 2
Ab Curl 2

Stretches -
Foot/Ankle/Leg Stretch
Quad/Hip Flexor Stretch
Forward Bend with Twist
Forward Bend
Mermaid
Spinal Twist 3

Weights:
Rotator Strengthener
Chest Fly
Lat Pullover

Band:
Inner Thigh Shaper
Incorporate resistance band into previously learned pilates

Ball:
Push Up
Buttock Firmer

Century Exercise

yuchea urlcheawee 유체 울체의 (fluid motion) 41-50

Meditation – Proper Attitude

Notes

Meaning: Earth; maturity, strength, & stability
              (Spiritually – stable in character & belief)

Tiger One Steps 10-11
Dragon One Steps 10-11

Balance – Lift one leg in a high front snap kick and hold for 60+ sec

Pilates -   Oblique Strengthener
               Sitting Pose Sequence
               Grande Ronde de Jambe
               Ballet Brush Front
               Teaser 1
               Roll Down 3
               T Stand 1
               Downward Facing Dog 1
               Plank 2
               Can-Can 2
               Rolling Like a Ball
               Low Hover 1

Stretches -   Lateral Spiral Stretch
               Lateral Stretch
               Warrior
               Open Leg Stretch

Weights -   Biceps Curl
               Standing Front Raise
               Chest Press

Ball -   Outer Hip and Thigh Slimmer
               Inner Thigh Firmer
               Ab/Torso Toner

Decade Exercise

yuchea urlcheawee 유체 울체의 (fluid motion) 51-60

Meditation – Proper Values

Notes

Meaning: Fire; source of warmth & earth's "blood flow"
                  (Spiritually – Christ's blood once accepted as salvation is source
                  of inner strength)

Tiger One Steps 12-13
Dragon One Steps 12-13

Balance – Lift leg straight back, lean forward with arms held out front of body in the
          dragon flight pose and hold for 60+ sec

Pilates -   Back Strengthener (on Knees)
                  Plank 3
                  Low Hover 2
                  Downward Facing Dog 2
                  Shoulder Stand 1
                  Leg Lift Reach 2
                  T Stand 2
                  Teaser 2

yuchea urlcheawee 유체 울체의 (fluid motion) 61-70

Push Hands – Basic

Meditation – all

Instructing Experience

Health and Diet – Nutritional Facts

Notes

Tiger One-Step Sparring

#1 –
- as attacker punches slide 45° to left, fighting stance
- at the same time perform a reverse outer block
- punch straight in to temple

#2 –
- as attacker punches slide 45° to left, fighting stance
- at the same time perform a outer block
- elbow strike to chin

#3 –
- as attacker punches slide 45° to left, fighting stance
- front kick to rib cage

#4 –
- as attacker punches slide 45° to left, fighting stance
- grab wrist
- turn back hip to hip and elbow strike to base of spinal column

#5 –
- as attacker punches slide 45° to left, fighting stance
- right side kick to rib cage
- tornado crescent kick

#6 –
- as attacker punches slide to fighting stance
- jump and at same time crescent kick to opponent's arm and thrust kick

#7 –
- double knife block
- twist
- push and pull backfist
- torque

#8 –
- step in and left outer block
- push and pull hammer fist
- step and sweep
- ridge hand take down

#9 –
- slide side back and palm block
- front round kick to knee
- moon thrust to knee
- flip

#10 –
- slide in to dragon stance
- left dragon block
- right dragon strike
- left dragon claw
- grab head
- step dragon punch

#11 –
- step in right to fighting stance
- double knife block
- double spear hand
- left jump back spin side kick

#12 –
- right step back
- left palm block
- left reverse round kick
- right back spin hook to head

#13 –
- left outer block
- push and pull
- right elbow strike
- jump left front kick

Notes

Notes

Dragon One-Step Sparring

\# 1 – against single hand grab

- trap hand
- twist
- front kick to underbelly

\# 2 – against single hand grab

- trap hand
- twist with help on elbow
- thrust kick to rib cage

\# 3 – against double hand grab

- trap
- grab both thumbs
- push down toward wrists
- knee strike to chin

\#4 – against head lock

- tuck chin
- drop weight and knock knee from behind
- push on back of hip and elbow

\#5 – against grab from behind

- grab appendage
- drop weight
- twist out
- lock arm

\#6 – against straight punch

- block
- flick nose or injung

\#7 – against punch

- right knife block
- left grab hand and twist out
- step in right elbow to neck
- step circle out throw with elbow

8 – against punch or grab

- step left and knife block – grab
- step right head lock holding hand
- snap neck
- small circle
- dragon reap (left take out legs – right throw body)

9 – against punch or grab

- basic block – take down
- side fall
- scissor legs
- dragon roll

10 – against punch or grab

- modified left dragon claw to inner elbow
- right moon thrust into left jump side kick

11 – against grab and punch
- palm heel lock/strike
- forearm strike neck of grabber
- step back leg closest to puncher
- bring both attacker down together
- lock punching arm around neck of other attacker

12 – against a high two handed grab
- Koreo block to:
wrist, right under elbow, right above triceps, and final strike to throat

13 – against a straight punch or stab
- step to the outside of the attacking arm
- scissor block similar to "creation" to break the elbow
- Finish – ideally roll over the back
swoop kick from other side to face or throat

Notes

Notes

Gibon Hana
- horse stance
- to solo plexus   left punch, right punch, left punch
- to injung   right punch, left punch, right punch
- to solo plexus   left inner block right punch, left punch
- to solo plexus   right inner block, left punch, right punch
- to solo plexus   left high block, right punch, left punch
- to solo plexus   right high block, left punch, right punch

Gibon Dul
- horse stance
- to injung, solo plexus   left knife strike, right punch, left punch
- to injung, solo plexus   right knife strike, left punch, right punch
- to solo plexus   left outer block, right punch, left punch
- to solo plexus   right outer block, left punch, right punch
- to solo plexus   right pressing down block, left spear hand, left back fist, right punch, left punch
- to solo plexus   left pressing down block, right spear hand, right back fist, left punch, right punch

Gibon Set
- ready stance   double outer block, double uppercut
- horse stance   fighting guard left, circle to top double knife down block
- horse stance   fighting guard right, circle to top double knife down block
- horse stance   double outer block, double uppercut, double down block
- ready stance   spreading block

Gibon Net
- horse stance
- to left   left outer block, left down block, left hammer fist
- to right   right outer block, right down block, right hammer fist
- left tiger stance   right palm block, right back fist
- left front stance   left punch right punch
- right tiger stance   left palm block, left back fist
- right front stance   right punch, left punch
- left back stance   left knife block
- left front stance   right elbow strike, right back fist, left punch
- right back stance   right knife block
- right front stance   left elbow strike, back fist, right punch

Notes

Pal chaggi Hana
- fighting stance
- repeat names of each kick on each set

⇑   right front kick, left front kick
⇓   left front kick, right side kick
⇑   right front kick, left round kick
⇓   left front kick, right crescent kick

Pal chaggi Dul
- fighting stance
- repeat "Shinsei Mu Sool" on each kick

⇑   right front kick, left front kick, right front kick
⇓   right front kick, left side kick, right side kick
⇑   right front kick, left round kick, right round kick
⇓   right front kick, left crescent kick, right crescent kick

Pal chaggi Set
- fighting stance
- repeat "Shinsei Mu Sool" on each kick

⇑   right front kick, left front kick, skip left front kick
⇓   left front kick, right side kick, skip right side kick
⇑   right front kick, left round kick, skip left round kick
⇓   left front kick, right crescent kick, skip right crescent kick

Notes

Notes

Notes

Notes

www.ingramcontent.com/pod-product-compliance
Lightning Source LLC
Chambersburg PA
CBHW041518280526
45792CB00004B/1296